"*Mood Blitz* is a realistic, yet triumphant book. Anyone reading this clearly and movingly written book will have a real understanding of, not only Bipolar Disorder, but the human condition. I give it my highest recommendation."

— Jeffrey C. Hutzler, MD
Distinguished Fellow, American Psychiatric Association
Cleveland Clinic Department of Psychiatry, retired

"An intimate look at what it is like to live with Bipolar illness, the good and the ugly. Marti writes with the same frenetic pace that she speaks and thinks. Sometimes you can almost sense how fast her mind works in her writing. I especially liked the chapter by her husband—it's nice to hear from both sides of the couple—one who is living it and one who is living with it. A candid portrayal of the life (so far) of someone who lives with bipolar disorder daily."

— Brad Berger, MD
Child, Adolescent and Adult Psychiatry
Adena Counseling Center, Chillicothe, Ohio

"Marti displays vulnerability and courage through the telling of her life with manic-depression. Sometimes heart warming, sometimes gritty and insane, this true-to-life tale gives wonderful insight into the struggles and accomplishments of one who tries to maximize the wellness in her life. As demonstrated in her story, the best ally in living with the reality of chronic illness is the awareness of the whole of your life. Marti lives in this awareness and encourages others to do so as well."

— Randal Blain
Psychiatric Chaplain, Barnes-Jewish Hospital
St. Louis, Missouri

"As someone diagnosed with bipolar over twenty years ago, I found *Mood Blitz* to be powerful and enlightening. The author has given me insights that will help me manage my illness in the future."

— Aubrey B.
Consumer

"It's impossible to fully comprehend what it's like to live with bipolar disorder, but Marti Markley's *Mood Blitz* provides a candid look at how her condition has affected every area of her life for forty years. From racing thoughts and insomnia to anxiety and depression, she covers a plethora of symptoms with humor and down-to-earth candor. If you only read one book on this subject, it should be *Mood Blitz*."

— Bobbi Linkemer
Author of *Words To Live By*
Reflections on the writing life from a 40-year veteran

Mood bLitz

Bipolar Disorder: An onslaught of Mania and Depression

Marti Markley

LinkUp
Publishing

Mood Blitz
Bipolar Disorder: An Onslaught of Mania and Depression
by Marti Markley

ISBN: 978-0-9826746-2-8
Library of Congress Control Number: 2010934169

Book designed by Nehmen-Kodner: www.n-kcreative.com
Printed in the United States of America

Published by LinkUp Publishing
www.moodblitz.com
marti@moodblitz.com

Dedication

For people with bipolar disorder,
their families, and the professionals
who treat them

CONTENTS

AcKNOWLEdgMENtS

I wish to thank my son, Jarek, for computer assistance and my daughter, Jeanine, for editing and writing support.

A special thanks to Bobbi Linkemer, my coach and mentor, for encouraging my writing efforts, even when I was facing a bipolar crisis.

I owe a debt of gratitude to my husband, who confronted my bipolar life and managed to remain strong.

Finally, I want to express gratitude and affection for the efforts my mother and father made in living with my bipolar condition and giving me hope that I could conquer it.

Preface

Most memoirs I've read by people with bipolar disorder begin with a crisis, possible suicidal tendencies, hospitalizations, and descriptions of the author's suffering. But after much experimentation with doctors, therapists, and medications, the author ultimately turns a corner and finds new ways of coping. Hope for the future becomes not only possible, but also attainable. In the process, the author becomes somewhat of a success story for prevailing over this debilitating condition.

My book does not follow this familiar pattern. It is about changes—in mood, lifestyle, medication, coping strategies—I have experienced in my life as a hostage to my bipolar condition for the last four decades. As a person with bipolar disorder, I have learned much about typical major stressors by reading memoirs that helped clarify the challenges caused by this mood disorder. Reading them has provided me with some comfort as I sought answers to my own difficult situation. I am grateful to the authors for sharing their personal and intimate accounts of a condition that often takes years to understand. In addition, textbooks and handbooks about bipolar disorder have provided comprehensive and valuable information.

Yet, in some ways my memoir is similar to others; it includes recollections of crises, medication trials, and suffering. These things go with the territory, so to speak. I, too, have experimented with different approaches with the help of medical people, counselors, and pharmaceuticals. I have turned a few corners now and then and definitely found new ways of coping with my illness. That's where the similarity stops.

To tell the truth, I have not prevailed, and sometimes my hope for the future wanes. Since I first became ill at the age of twelve, my life has been pretty much an unstable ride. Positive periods do occur—times when I resume my ability to do such things as working part-time, playing piano, exercising, meeting with friends.

In these last forty years, every aspect of my life has been affected by bipolar disorder. I have experienced major mood swings, dramatic fluctuations in energy, and all kinds of physical ailments that have affected my family life, career, how I relate to others and make major life decisions ... even my decision about whether to have a family. Sometimes I have so much energy, I overextend myself physically and crash; other times, I am weak and unable to motivate myself to get off the couch. Sometimes I am boisterous and apparently amusing; at the other extreme, I am anxious, irritable, and hopeless.

There is no question that modern medicine has made great strides in treating this illness, but unfortunately not everyone with bipolar disorder has a happily-ever-after story to share. For some of us, the struggle is continuous. A medication may work for a while, then quit. Or a new set of symptoms may present itself, and the search for the proper drug begins anew.

I am one of those people who have never hit a permanent plateau. When I feel well, I try to live my life as normally as possible; when I don't, I have learned to listen to my body. My husband is supportive, though I don't think he is entirely able to understand the disorder or what I am experiencing. Fortunately, he's a positive person, or this would have been even harder on our family than it has been.

Patty Duke did all of us a great favor when she wrote her memoir, *A Brilliant Madness*. She shed light on a subject that had been kept in the shadows for far too long. Current memoir writers follow her brave example. We write to help others who have bipolar disorder; to educate families, the public, and the medical profession; and to put an end to the stigma associated with mental illness. I believe that is our obligation and our privilege.

Racing after talking, moving,
don't constrain me.

Fragmented mind, loss,
I can't bypass my mind.

Depression always coexsists,
seething below the surface
or smacks me in the head.

The bipolar course
persists relentlessly.

— Marti Markley

1 BipoLar TaLK

I have bipolar disorder, which is another term for manic-depression. It is the diagnosis that includes both depression and mania. Depression symptoms include depressed mood, loss of ability to feel pleasure, social withdrawal, suicidal thoughts, poor concentration, fatigue, sleep disturbances, and insomnia. Manic symptoms—quite the opposite—comprise elation, euphoria, increased energy and libido, decreased need for sleep, racing thoughts, and irritable mood. I will often mention hypomania. The distinction between mania and hypomania is one of severity. A person with hypomania has a high level of energy, resulting in more ideas, creativity, and productivity. Although some people feel good during the hypomanic phase, many do not and experience irritability, agitation, and an inability to discern reality. Mania is further along that continuum and usually includes distorted thinking and the psychotic features of hallucinations and delusions.

A person with bipolar disorder may experience overlaps (mixed states) between depression and mania. Of course, I didn't learn this until many years after my symptoms began.

As chaotic as these conditions are individually, they may overlap or cycle rapidly. Of course, I didn't learn this until many years after my symptoms began. When depression and mania overlap, my positive mood is gone, and I feel disabled and dysphoric. Rapid cycling, which I have experienced many times, is defined as four or more episodes of depression cycling to mania or mania to depression occurring within one year. These unexpected and frequent mood swings have made my condition difficult to treat because my drug regimen needs to be quickly reevaluated.

In the early days of my condition, not only were there no medications, there was no diagnosis. Thankfully, that situation has changed. The new drugs for bipolar disorder allow us to cope with our chaotic and challenging lives. I think it is essential for anyone with bipolar to realize that medications actually work on bipolar pathways or transmitters in the brain. Depression is a sign of reduced serotonin or norepinephrine transmitters. Mania is the opposite—a case of too many transmitters. These chemicals have been mystifying researchers and doctors for many years. But now, studies of chemicals linked to bipolar brains have led to pharmaceutical trials and the creation of new drugs—the salvation of people like me. Mood-stabilizing and antidepressant drugs do work for most people, and each decade we can look forward to new drugs to improve our lives.

The drugs are improving every year, and it is likely that a good match can be found between a bipolar person's brain chemicals and the various drugs on the market.

When people talk about bipolar disorder, they are usually referring to the mental diagnosis, but I have found there is a physical component as well. After all, my mind and body are connected; living with bipolar is essentially a mind-body experience. Sometimes my body works fine, and other times my mind does. But sometimes my physical and mental sides are both having problems. Throughout my life, these extremes have seemed to chase me, and I have done what I could to outrun them.

Technically, I know that bipolar disorder is all about moods, but the description of a mood seems so fleeting and shallow compared with the depth of the episodes people experience. It is not just happy or sad moods but a pervasive depression/mania that affects all parts of one's existence.

I refer to an *episode* to mean an intense period, either manic or depressive, lasting a few weeks or months. Usually, I bottom out and become debilitated enough that my previous treatment is not working well. Then, I need something new—a medication change from my psychiatrist to fix me and bring me out of my slump.

When I first experienced this illness, no one seemed to be able to figure out what was wrong with me. Before 1973, there were few drugs to help me cope. Taking the newer drugs, juggling medications, and being patient with myself—yet assertive with medical professionals—are some of the ways I have learned to confront this overpowering disorder.

At this point, there is no cure; there are only ways to tame and balance all those mysterious chemicals and symptoms when they flare up. So, that's what I do. Sometimes, it's a full-time job.

Depression: A mental state characterized by a pessimistic sense of inadequacy, sad feelings of gloom, and a despondent lack of activity

I was at a high school
basketball game with a
friend when depression
first hit.

It was like my head dropped
to the floor and I was
scared to move.

I was so confused I could
not find my way out of the
auditorium.

— Marti Markley

2 My Twelve-Year-Old Crisis

My illness began abruptly and for no reason when I was twelve. It was a dramatic episode of hideous and painful depression and corresponding mania. It felt like a great force was trying to annihilate me. I lived in a dark hole, while pervasive anxiety and agitation of my mind and body would not let me rest. From the beginning, I struggled to keep above the surface, to reach the sky and sun—my only hope. But the water turned dark and the sky and sun were unattainable. Actually, *I* was the dark one, and I was leaving the world behind me. Depression deranged my life and shut out any happiness. This was the beginning of my bipolar odyssey.

My catastrophe seemed an accident, soon to be fixed, I was sure. My life was a mystery. Nothing in my environment, my conscious or subconscious life, seemed to have caused this. For months, I had no appetite and could not sleep well. I awoke each night at two or three A.M. and watched the clock move. As seconds became hours, I lay there with fear ravaging my heart and adrenaline flowing through me, wondering *why*? As I recall, those painful hours lasted for years. I entertained thousands of negative thoughts during my sleepless nights. I longed for the simple and happy past when sleep obliterated the seconds on a clock. Maybe I should never have had a clock in my bedroom.

> *My life was a mystery. Nothing in my environment, my conscious or subconscious life, seemed to have caused this.*

The depression chemicals were changing my ability to do simple jobs. One day, my mother asked me to sweep the porch. I took the broom from her hand but could not figure out how to use it. My mind was twisted and confused. Small tasks had become insurmountable. My mother ushered me outside. Where should I sweep the debris? For a half hour, I moved slowly, started to sweep, turned around, and started to sweep again. I didn't remember whether I had swept the porch. I felt guilty. I was handicapped.

Since I was rapid cycling every few days or weeks, my mood fluctuated wildly, but my mother had learned to tell exactly how I was feeling by such clues as my posture and facial expressions. She was the only person who guessed about my depression. She watched me walk down our quiet street to see if my head was bowed. That's how she knew I was in a depressed phase.

I cried for hours each day and was either too tired or too agitated and fearful to start an activity. My mother listened to me rant and rave, hoping to problem solve the depression. Undoubtedly, my siblings received little attention during my mood changes. But I didn't have any reason to cry; nothing had changed in my life. Since I had only recently experienced my first "breakdown," I still remembered being healthy and could not accept my present condition.

Making mountains out of molehills was my perpetual problem, according to my dad. He explained his very simple philosophy to me several times during my childhood because I had occasional anxiety episodes, and I didn't have a clue what to do about them. The idea is to avoid exaggerating a situation and making a big deal (mountain) out of a small problem (molehill). If I could do this, I would relax and find reality, he told me. But, if I had been more dramatic or more panicky, I might have landed in the hospital, and perhaps someone could have diagnosed my problem. Instead, I was sitting right out in the open, a sitting duck for the next round of depression.

My hometown was a small Midwestern one with big, old houses and tree-lined streets. It was built around agriculture, railroads, and a small college. The stability was good, and it was very safe. I could walk downtown in twenty minutes and go to the movies or to the high school. In eighteen years, we had never seen a traffic jam. It was a friendly, ordinary place. Besides me, there was only one other girl we knew of in our town who was also depressed.

Psychiatrists and psychologists were called in each year of my young life, beginning at age twelve, to probe for a diagnosis and treatment. However, no one seemed to understand bipolar or "manic-depression." Before I graduated from college, I had experienced two state hospital professionals, a Freudian psychiatrist, two private-practice psychologists, and a university counselor. I received some excellent counseling that, frankly, would have helped anyone. I gained confidence and learned that coping was staying above the turbulent waters and fighting to clear my head of chaos. This proved to be an immense job, with no help in 1966 from pharmaceutical drugs to tame my own chemicals.

Before Bipolar

My life before bipolar had been good. I was motivated and talented in sports, music, and art. I liked school and playing with friends. I was outgoing, sensitive, and energetic. In my family, I was the most emotional and probably the most intense.

At four, I was known as tough and happy. I was always on the go and moved quickly. My mother remembers placing me in preschool so that I could channel my energies. My artistic talent developed at preschool. In class, I would be the first one to finish my picture, which enabled me to be the "policeman" on the playground. My teacher would usually mumble something like, "Well, you can't be done. Let me see your picture. Oooh, this is excellent! You can go outside." Painting and drawing were like walking for me, and I liked being the policeman because I could boss around all the boys. At home, I had to struggle to get this power over my three brothers.

Psychiatrists and psychologists were called in each year of my young life, beginning at age twelve.

By age eight, I was still extroverted and athletic but developed a need to conform and became overly conscientious at school. This anxiety continued throughout grade school. I was a tough ball player and had close friends, but I began to get depressed during bad weather. If dark clouds lasted more than one day, I instantly got in a bad mood. When the sun came out, I was ecstatic.

I was very sensitive to my surroundings and to people and would often feel pain if someone else was hurt. My mother would tell me it was OK to feel pain for others and for myself because it made me more aware of life. I spent a lot of time with my dad, planting in the garden and going with him on calls to see his clients. We shared an outlook and relaxed communication that were so similar, we could understand each other without speaking more than a few words. We were both highly intuitive and liked to have fun.

But at twelve, I was a confused preadolescent who was trapped with oppressive, raging brain chemicals and no ability to fix myself. My life had changed drastically. My hope was in our family and in the medical world. My family was strong, persistent, and open-minded, always looking for new ways to handle situations. I trusted my parents completely; I knew they would help me out of this mess. My parents were as shocked by my depression as I was. (We did not know I was depressed at the time.) Each day, they listened as I tried to tell them about my reality. They became very sad because they thought they were losing me. It is hard to say whether my parents suffered more than I did. Looking back, I would say they did. To me, everyone looked very strong. I could not see their suffering through my own.

Sweet Thirteen

My loving grandparents always visited for my birthday dinner, and the thirteenth was special to them. "You are no longer a child and will soon be a young lady," my grandma said, and that was enough. I had already heard these puberty-related remarks from the neighbors, but I refused to accept that "womanhood talk." Did they forget I was the neighborhood tomboy and that Peter Pan and I were fierce deniers? I didn't need to grow up. Besides, I was depressed; my head was heavy; I could barely carry it around; and I didn't want to eat a delicious meal or birthday cake. I tried to concentrate, constantly, on all the ways I was supposed to fit in at each occasion. Today was not one of them. I asked my mom if I could please be excused to go to my room because I was suffocating. She said yes.

Everyone agreed that I had to struggle with reality and *cope.* School was torture. I couldn't concentrate, and I was sad and anxious. I had so many thoughts tumbling around in my mind: Don't say this; don't do that; do the math problem; don't get up until everyone leaves; don't let them know I've changed; act normal. All I wanted was to go to bed.

I had two loyal friends, both named Mary, who came to my house one day after school. They had noticed the change in my behavior and were cautious in communicating with me. They thought I was being a snob because I was distant with everyone and didn't do anything with people anymore. They said I might start losing some of my friends. This was how depression appeared to them. I felt guilty in one way and angry in another. What had I done to these friends? I knew they didn't have a clue about my mental health. I said something like "whatever" when they left my house. I was hopeless. I couldn't be a warm human being. I couldn't laugh, I couldn't enjoy them anymore, and I couldn't change my social situation.

When I was fifteen, my father pulled me aside one day. He had on his serious face, which was rare for him, so I listened.

"Your counseling can give you a great advantage," he said. "You will know yourself better, be more confident, and be able to cope with your life. I haven't experienced counseling," he admitted, "and neither has anyone in our family, except for you."

I was struck with the enormity of this observation and was already beginning to notice changes in myself.

Now, thinking back forty years after many years of counseling, I know my dad was right, and I'm glad. I got his message early enough to realize it is difficult to understand ourselves. Counseling helps us see many new dimensions of our lives. It gives us insight that lasts a lifetime.

Rapid cycling: Multiple episodes of depression and mania within a given year; changes in mood from mania to major depression, or mixed states, within hours, days, or months

Psychiatrists are vital in the
therapeutic process to carefully
monitor and treat ever-changing
mood swings.

As astute patients, we can begin
therapy by interviewing
our psychiatrists to see
if their methods meet our needs.

Asking pertinent questions
is important.

— Marti Markley

3 Psychiatrists, Psychologists, and Treatments

My depression took many forms over the years; in my early years from twelve to sixteen, it was dark and powerful. I also switched over to a hypomanic state every few weeks or months. When that happened, I felt much improved, very confident, physically energetic, and somewhat euphoric. My parents were always glad to see me this way! My brain felt liberated, and I knew I could function in this mode indefinitely.

I did not get a diagnosis of bipolar until I was twenty-three, so I spent a lot of time in therapy.

The following discussion of psychiatrists, psychotherapists, and therapies demonstrates the only direction I knew for ten years. I did not get a diagnosis of bipolar until I was twenty-three, so I spent a lot of time in talk therapy. Before I was twenty-three, few bipolar-specific drugs were available; lithium was one of the few. I was never hospitalized because, somehow, I could appear to be functioning well; and I was compliant with the doctors. The reason I went along with my parents' ideas about therapists was that they were convincing, and they knew the medical field. What I knew was that I was hanging on by a thread, so I would try anything.

Looking back, I know that therapy helped me to cope with my life and always seemed to straighten out my problems.

My overall experience with psychiatrists and psycho-therapists was intriguing and safe. Looking back, I know that therapy helped me to cope with my life and always seemed to straighten out my problems. However, in my body and in my mind, I still had bipolar disorder; the chemicals had not changed. I needed medications, but I didn't know they existed.

Now, psychiatric sessions are about twenty minutes long; they used to be an hour. Over the years, I have learned to bring my notes and discuss my issues. The better my notes, the more topics we can discuss. Until next week or next month or the months after that, all I have to do is write notes. That's my job. Of course, I do have to remember any new regimen or lifestyle changes the psychiatrist suggests.

I have had twelve psychiatrists and psychotherapists in four states over forty years. Here is a rundown on who they were and how I responded to them.

Starting the Journey

My parents knew the medical director of the Illinois state mental facility, and my dad asked him to come over to meet me. It was after my initial break, so I was in pieces—depressed and unsure about what to do. Frankly, I couldn't have made a decision if I had tried. However, my mother mentioned that I actually *was* functioning on some level, since I was still going to school.

I remember that year in school as absolute torture, when I spent a lot of time hanging out in the bathroom to escape my teachers. Eventually, my teacher caught me, and she was very sensitive to my needs. She called my mom, who picked me up from school. All of a sudden, the subject matter in my classes was extremely difficult. Everything was difficult. So, at this interview with the doctor, which would be the first of many interviews I would sit through to help them understand what kind of nonsense was going on in my brain, I was numb. I remember being in a fog, not knowing how to answer his questions. He asked me to meet with one of his best counselors and take some tests. I agreed because I knew I had no alternative.

I was so desperate, I would do anything. At age twelve I had to relinquish my ego and conform to the wishes of my parents, counselors, and doctors.

At that point, the staff doctors discussed with my parents the possibility of my admission to the hospital. They said, however, that I wouldn't fit in. The other kids would overpower me, and I probably wouldn't benefit. I was petrified to imagine living in the state facility, but they knew I was sick enough to be in the hospital. The major reason was the depression, even though I was also having extreme hypomanic episodes. The alternative was counseling. My parents were familiar with the counseling process, and they thought I should give it a chance. It was my best option at that time.

1. Psychologist • 1966 • Illinois

My first psychologist was a very sophisticated, intelligent woman who tried to stabilize me and make my depression less hideous. She had an impossible job. We worked hard together, and I liked her. She was eager to delve into my personality, which was usually dark, scared, negative, and oppressed. She was positive and realistic. She talked quietly and hinted at directions I could think about because my mind was often racing and not paying attention. I listened to her, and her messages sank in.

She helped me understand my parents—their demands, their personalities, their basic effect on me—and how to assert myself. Dealing with brothers and sisters was included in the package. We often walked through the grounds of the state facility and to the commissary. We took our time. We didn't rush. My counselor wanted to introduce me to a more casual way of living, since I was so uptight and such a perfectionist. We did some relaxation exercises—at least I tried to, but I was too anxiety-ridden. It was pathetic.

My first psychologist talked quietly and hinted at actions I should think about. Then she would repeat her ideas each session because my mind was often racing and not paying attention.

At the beginning, my bipolar was wild, with two or three weeks of depression followed by a switch to hypomania for a week or two. During the depressions, I listened very carefully to my counselor to see how I could get out of my mess. When I switched to hypomania, I always told the counselor that she created my magic switch. She told me, no, *I* had made the change. I was looking for cause and effect. But bipolar is volatile and erratic. Something inside me was twisting me in two directions.

She put me through advanced level "coping skills." She made me understand I could move on in life. This was a big idea for me. So, my first counseling experience was a great success; however, there was no talk of diagnosis. After a year and a half, my counselor took another job, and I was saddened. I had an unusual but safe relationship with her. I always knew she cared for me and wanted me to get better.

2. Psychiatrist • 1967 • Illinois

My second mental health professional also worked at the state hospital, but as a psychiatrist, not a psychotherapist. She treated the heavy-duty patients and was always very distracted, running around trying not to give in to the patients' demands, such as cigarettes, candy, and privileges. She tried to figure me out, briefly, and then asked me to do math problems. Math was not my favorite topic, but she had me do simple problems, ones I could easily answer. She thought this was a big deal and started asking me factual questions about our world, like who the president was, the name of my school, and what my classes were. I never figured out her angle.

I told her at the beginning of our sessions about my depression, how it took over my life, and how miserable and insecure I was. I felt as if I had to prove some wacko sickness to her. Here, I was conversing intelligently with her and being logical but depressed at the same time. At that time, I was still having major sleep disturbances, crying, feeling worthless, becoming detached from my friends, losing weight, and having difficulty concentrating. I was unable to imagine the future.

I don't think she understood about kids' depression. Maybe all the depressed kids in my town were staying home. I know I was not unique. Had I been a druggie or violent or a runaway, she would have been serious about a therapeutic plan. When I was thirteen, we moved on, but for many months we didn't know whom to turn to. I am so glad my parents understood that the disease I had was not cool and that *somewhere* there had to be help for me.

3. Psychiatrist • 1967 • Illinois

My parents were referred to a Freudian psychiatrist, and we traveled a good distance to see him. It was 1967, and I was thirteen. He was a nice person but seemed perplexed about how to handle me. I was having the same depression I started with, but he did not see this. Like other doctors, he said I was stable, everything was OK, and, what was I doing in his office? I remember telling him about my symptoms, which were really the classic symptoms of depression. He didn't appear to hear me. I remember thinking his approach was bizarre. He didn't seem to be in touch with his own reality, let alone mine.

I did not like lying on his couch. Why couldn't I sit up in a chair so we could look at each other's faces? I expected him to ask me weird questions about my life, but the questions were about how I related to the universe and other loosely strung-together philosophical topics. It seemed as if we were doing a science experiment.

With each visit, I got more confused. It wasn't counseling, and it wasn't psychiatry because there wasn't any medicine. The sessions were wearing me down. My diagnosis was "super sensitive." I told my parents how weird the situation was, as I fully described each visit to them. We made our exit. I wasn't laughing, then. I am now.

4. Psychologist • 1969 • Illinois

In 1969, a new psychologist, a PhD, moved into our small town and set up private practice. My depression had lifted somewhat, but rapid cycling was still a problem. Although I had learned to cope better with my depression, it didn't go away. This new psychotherapist was not very keen on treating my depression. You'd think he would have offered me something, such as an herbal remedy or vitamins. In my opinion, it seemed as though the psychiatric community must have really been confused about how to help a depressed adolescent, so they waited for the pharmaceutical industry to develop the drugs to deal with the problem.

By this time, I was ready to tell a counselor anything. Part of me was very outgoing. We talked a lot. He knew a lot about people, and I listened to him. I was beginning junior high school, trying to survive. I think he understood my basic insecurities as a teenager and set up a plan for my growth, while assessing my strengths and weaknesses. At this time, I was mostly hypomanic and less depressed, so I was having some fun.

My parents transferred me from Catholic school to the public school in eighth grade. I began with great hope for the possibilities of diverse classes and a larger student body. I was unstable but determined to keep myself mainstreamed. Many kids welcomed me, and, since my mental health secret was intact, the school year was looking good.

In high school, I began to experience mixed states. I remember being depressed in art class, which was probably my best subject. I was afraid of everyone and had to plan what to say if I was going to talk at all. I knew people could see through me. I was very serious and tried to look as if I knew what I was doing. When I slowed down at times, I became very irritable. I was known for being hyperactive, so I was doing a good job of hiding my symptoms. The class lasted forever each day. I always got recognition for my work, but most of the time I couldn't connect mentally to the pencil I was drawing with. My head felt like a mushroom.

Fortunately, at this point a true friend came along. Katrina, whom I met in class, was like me: sensitive, smart, talented, invisible to the social scene, not yet blooming, and stuck in a rut. Together, we had an enormous amount of fun on her farm and at school. She boosted my confidence and talked with me about my intimate problems. We both desired recognition from other classmates, so we learned to express ourselves and become competent adolescents. It was a lot of work, but we were determined.

I continued with the fourth therapist; it was nice to know that I could always land at his office, which I needed to do continuously because I was still untreated and feeling depressed or anxious to varying degrees most of the time.

However, I was learning how to deal with parents and friends. None of my friends was getting the insight I was gaining; nonetheless, I wasn't sure it was cool to go to a counselor. I think I stayed in the closet for ten years! I was getting the message that it was totally up to me to keep myself together. People thought I was capable, and, although I didn't think so, I kept coping. It was like a giant puzzle for which I had to find a few more pieces each year to add to the picture.

I was getting ready to go to college in 1972, and I was excited but somewhat scared. By this time, though, I was starting to accept myself as being botched up.

My college years were a mixture of hypomanic and depressed moods; however, I enjoyed my classes and friends. Overall, these years were very productive for me. I didn't seek any professional help during that time.

5. Mental Health Counselor • 1977 • Colorado

My fifth counselor worked in a clinic in Evergreen, Colorado. I had just graduated from the University of Denver, and, of course, my major was psychology. I was always surrounded by psych this and psych that. My motivation for seeking a counselor this time was to help me figure out my relationship with a guy I'd been dating for five years. We did not communicate well, and, even though I put a lot of energy into the relationship, I felt that he was not cooperating. Over time, I became angry and unstable. I was a wreck.

My first appointment was with a woman who had only her bachelor's degree. She was good because she was very intuitive, focused on what I said, and made it easy for me to express my thoughts. I remember looking out the big glass windows in her office at the mountains and pine trees. It was a very relaxing place. She helped me with the relationship, and in two weeks I was pulling away from my boyfriend, fast. But meanwhile, I was angry, crying, and quick to explode.

One day, I wadded Kleenex into balls and threw them all over her office. Of course, I was screaming and pounding my fists, too. She let me do all this and then reported my behavior to her boss. They thought I could be manic-depressive. This was what I had wished for all my life: a diagnosis! She also thought I might become violent.

I was shocked, but I was also relieved. I had waited for this day for ten years. I was ready to let people with knowledge manage my life. Apparently, I had not been able to do it because my brain chemicals were running amok. I really liked the idea that my brain chemicals were messing up of their own accord and that I wasn't to blame.

At first, I was numb. What kind of disease was this? Then, I realized I knew everything about this disease. It had consumed me; I consumed it. Next, I thought, what if some medications really worked? I was sure *something* good would happen to me. Of course, I did not realize that lithium had been around for only a few years. What I know now is that at twenty-three I began scrutinizing drugs—a practice I would continue for the rest of my life, seeing if they would work, gambling.

It turns out there was no single drug to heal all. Nobody would tell me how the medication game is played. It was like playing Monopoly, one square at time, one year at a time. And, then, sometimes you have to go to jail.

A doctor I saw twice prescribed my new drug treatment. He ordered 300 mg of lithium, three times a day. After taking it for a few days, I was vomiting, had diarrhea, and could barely move. I kept trying the same dose for three weeks and finally told the doctor it didn't work. Next, some genius figured out that I should take *one* 300 mg dose a day. Bingo.

I didn't rush around doing too many things at once. I felt tranquilized but not tired. A major area of my brain was settling down. I learned a drug approach that I would tell all future psychiatrists: Give me a small dose first. Then, we'll talk.

No Counselor • 1980 • California

Two years later, I moved to California after getting married to my husband, Evan. I admit my big mistake was not seeking help when I got there. I saw no reason to see a psychiatrist, so I floated along without support. Eventually, I became depressed and highly stressed to the point that I was taking sick leave. With constant headaches and irritable colon, I was having difficulty functioning. My marriage was, oddly enough, very stable and fun. Wow, was I lucky! But at work, I felt frozen and unable to fit in.

I was in the wrong job, but I felt compelled to keep working. The job was science-related, but I am naturally more artistically oriented. I remember feeling pressured by the competitive atmosphere and aware that I was losing ground. This was a source of constant frustration. I had to be responsible for myself because no friends or family really knew what was going on inside my brain. It took a great deal of time to explain myself to others, and I was not going to get any tips from anyone.

We moved from California to Ohio two years later, mainly to afford a home. Evan found a new job, and I was in transition, ready to change fields. We arrived in a snowstorm, which lasted forever, and there was no sun.

Everything was dark and oppressive. I must have sun! I didn't realize how sensitive I was to dark days. I was depressed and getting worse with each passing day.

Actually, I had been depressed for years but didn't know it. I didn't check in with a doctor because I didn't understand. I was still taking one lithium tablet per day, and I thought lithium should be my only drug. Then, I developed unexpected pain, which affected my back, fingers, legs, arms, and head. It was so hideous, and everyone thought I was weird. I went to a neurologist, who put me in the hospital for six days. The diagnosis was nerve-ending pain; the prescription was Elavil. It worked.

6. Psychiatrist • 1982 • Ohio

Next, I was referred to a psychiatrist at the Ohio State University Medical Center. Yes, he thought I was depressed; and, yes, he would start giving me more Elavil. It would save me for the time being. Besides being keen on drugs, my new psychiatrist was able to do a nice job of counseling me on my family, my conflicts, and my side effects. He was able to combine talk therapy and drug therapy, while being compassionate and intuitive in assessing my needs. I have seen many psychiatrists, as people with bipolar disorder do, but he easily excelled as perhaps the best.

7. Psychiatrist • 1984 • St. Louis

Before I moved to St. Louis, the clinic at Ohio State University gave me names of three good psychiatrists. Naturally, I did not see a doctor as soon as I moved because I felt invincible, all knowing, and in no need of someone to tell me how to live my bipolar life. But I waited too long, and mania crept into my system and caused me weeks of anguish. Finally, I accepted being out of control and contacted a female psychiatrist who suggested excellent changes in medication. She discussed my drugs and their properties, which I found extremely helpful. She also made herself available if I needed extra appointments. Within the next year, a depression occurred, and we juggled drugs. Once again, I had found a capable psychiatrist and could feel safe and secure.

8. Psychiatrists • 1991 • St. Louis

After six years, I believed that I needed a new doctor. I went online to find two doctors at a psychiatric facility that was listed through my health insurance plan. My experiences were not good at this facility. Patients typically waited one and a half hours every visit; there were only a few chairs in the waiting room; the waiting room was dirty; and there was no contact with office personnel. In treatment, my comments were often disregarded. Looking back, I see that finding a doctor through my health insurance plan was not as good as getting a direct referral. Finding a doctor takes time, and doing research is almost always necessary.

9. Psychiatrist • 2003 • St. Louis

After my eighth experience, I was able to get a referral for a new psychiatrist in St. Louis who really helped me with my mood disorder; he also had a sense of humor, which made my sessions with him enjoyable. He gained my trust by his empathetic nature and his straightforward, practical treatment approach. After three years, I was very sorry to see him move to Ohio.

10. Family-Care Practitioner • 1994 – present • St. Louis

My family-care practitioner has always been ready to fix whatever problems still remained after my visits to a psychiatrist. If a minor condition arose and I had no clue as to its origin, after a visit with him I would quickly see a new option. Once, I went off one tablet of antianxiety medication and was experiencing extreme agitation from the withdrawal. My family-care practitioner gave me a timetable of six weeks to go off the drug gradually. And it worked.

11. Psychiatrist • 2007 • St. Louis

My current psychiatrist steadfastly works to understand the best treatment for her patients. We have experimented systematically throughout several years. My appointments are generally spaced two to four weeks apart to accommodate my frequent mood swings. When my medications are stable, I "graduate" to a schedule of appointments once every three months. I have made this transition only twice in the past few years. I have full confidence that I am moving in the right direction.

I currently take a mix of antidepressants and mood stabilizers.

LIFE IS MY COLLEGE.

—ANONYMOUS

4 COLLEgE YEars aNd BEYONd

1972 – 1976 • *University of Denver*

M y college years at the University of Denver were a great break for me. I didn't have a major depression, and I had enough energy to complete my classes and projects. I felt good enough to start setting goals and began to believe in a future. I had bad days, but I don't remember them, for some reason. I just remember blue skies with forever sunshine and mountains. This interim period, which lasted about three years, was proof that bipolar disorder *is* capable of letting up, occasionally.

High school and college were easier to cope with than my very early depression years, when I was twelve to sixteen. I'm not sure why I chose a college 1,000 miles away from my parents, who were my support system. I realized that I could become a basket case at any time, but then a little denial is necessary to move forward. I just wanted a life, and I didn't care if I felt miserable part of the time. I was looking for positive experiences. So, my parents and I drove from Illinois to Denver, Colorado. I was excited to get started. I remember being extremely anxious, too, but I could handle it. I had a great roommate in my freshman year, which helped my stability.

Every day I viewed the mountains from my dorm window, and they became my spirituality, my happiness. My free time was devoted to getting into the mountains, although I didn't have a car. I loved the high altitude, the rivers, the huge boulders, the extreme-colored skies, and the mountain panoramas. One great feature of Denver is that it has many days of sunshine, especially in the winter. This helped my mood and kept me free of seasonal affective disorder (SAD). *See Chapter 10, SAD.*

During my first years in college I was hypomanic, but I stayed within my limits, so no one really noticed any unusual behavior. I was hyper and spacey and a bit wild. When I really felt great, I would dance down the halls in a free-form style that confused people who didn't know if I was a real dancer or just flying around. I usually made good decisions and kept myself motivated in my courses. I guess that's what kept me in college.

My emotional life was dependent upon my new friends. None of us had family within 1,000 miles, so we created new families in our dorm or our classes. I found a great friend, Sarah, who was liberal, as I was; we talked for hours about world topics and what we wanted to do with our lives. We were trying so hard to find the answers to life's questions and to fit into society. For every great thought we shared, we also had loads of fun goofing around. I found Sarah relaxed, which was good for me. She remained my best friend throughout college. Those years were also for boyfriends. What a racket—moving from one to the next, then spending months without anyone.

Every day I viewed the mountains from my dorm window, and they became my spirituality, my happiness.

My small group of friends occasionally experimented with drugs. They believed I was naturally high (and envied my condition), so they kept drugs out of my hands. They couldn't have known that drugs might have sent me in dangerous directions. I didn't know, either. They just gave me a beer or Coca-Cola and watched me get just as high as they were. I never got a chance to thank them for their intuition.

I met Jon when I was nineteen. He had just moved to Colorado from Chicago where he had been a disc jockey. He was an excellent singer and photographer. He also had a photographic memory. We seemed compatible and loved each other very much. I was able to see him only on the weekends because he lived in Evergreen.

None of us had family within 1,000 miles, so we created new families in our dorm or our classes.

For the first two years, our relationship was smooth. But then, reality set in. I was really concerned about his career and mine. He was twenty-four, and, since he was a few years older than I was, I felt he should be establishing himself professionally. I was very vocal in our arguments, probably out of control. Anything would set me off. In the fourth year of our relationship, the bipolar disorder was making me tired and irritable. My sleep was lousy most of the time. I was on edge.

We enjoyed living in Colorado and took every trip imaginable. We were very close for five years, although we had separations. I always wanted to move forward, but he was in denial about many issues in his life, including his career. Even when we talked about these issues, I felt Jon did not care about changing. Then, I would get frustrated, and he would escape into his music. I didn't think our future goals were compatible, and I was getting tired of spending so much time on the relationship.

I was desperate to talk to someone about Jon. I wasn't sleeping and couldn't focus on anything. I felt as if I had a rock inside my head. I couldn't relax. I was twenty-one and at the University of Denver when I contacted student counseling. Their services were free, just right for my budget. The woman I met with listened well and gave her real opinions, which I appreciated. Somehow, I knew that I would have to use my own powers to calm down; for people with bipolar, that was usually impossible.

My emotional life was dependent upon my new friends. .

I took from her what I could and got ready to make more life decisions. I felt more confident, even though I was messed up. I was hypomanic, at least, but she didn't label me. It is odd that a label, a diagnosis, would have been refreshing after eight years of self-discovery.

1976 • 22 years old

I had just graduated from the University of Denver with a major in psychology. Eventually, I realized that I was over-whelmed with psychology and psychiatry and decided to get out of this field because it was claustrophobic.

So, I started looking for jobs while experiencing poverty and feeling panicked. I had practically no contacts, but I wanted to remain in the Denver area. Every day, I wrote in a notebook the names of three contacts to pursue, like a to-do list. I made myself follow up on each entry. At the end of the day, I relaxed and allowed myself to do activities for fun or to be with friends without any guilt until the sun rose the next day. Job-hunting may be the most stressful activity ever. It always felt so degrading to me to be looking for a job when I wasn't really confident but had to appear as if I were.

Finally, I got a call from a woman who worked in a nursing home and wondered whether I was interested in a position as a social services representative. This job was perfect for me, as I was able to develop the program using my ideas and coordinate social services with the state of Colorado. I found that I loved working with the elderly population, and it was a great job for two and a half years.

I had ups and downs and insomnia during this period. I kept a daily chart on which I wrote a plus or a minus sign. The plus meant my head was fairly relaxed, but minus meant I had an irritable, hypomanic day. Sometimes, a good sleep would break a pattern of a negative cycle. My head was far from being stabilized.

In the meantime, the relationship with Jon was getting out of control again. It was one year after college, and things were continuing to deteriorate. I spent so much energy trying to communicate with him but never felt he matched my willingness to talk about our problems. I was at the end of a five-year relationship I had hoped would last forever. I was angry, so I stole some photos from him because he wouldn't share them with me. I wanted something to show for all the places we had traveled, mainly pictures of mountain sites.

Next, I decided to make a "presentation" for him, similar to the ones he made for clients, combining music and words. I spent several hours taping music to go along with dialogue I had for him focusing on our relationship—what it was and what it had become. It was a good presentation, but he never mentioned it to me. I knew the relationship couldn't continue. Love is torture.

1978 • 24 years old

I had a new boyfriend; his name was Evan. He was a friendly person, didn't worry about very much, and was seriously involved in his career in hydrogeology. I was attracted to him for those characteristics. I believe he liked my sense of humor and my energy, and we generally agreed on big topics in life—ethics, money, and morals. We both enjoyed being outdoors together. Neither of us was expecting a serious relationship, but after nine months, we just knew we would solidify our life together.

I told Evan I had bipolar two months after I met him. He was interested in this unique disease and was always asking me questions. I guess his head was so stable that he didn't mind a person with bipolar hanging around. He asked what he could do to help. This was the best question because I knew he would try to help me if he could.

The most difficult times for me were when I was depressed and tried to have someone understand that. The only way to understand depression is by experiencing it firsthand—actually being depressed. I knew Evan had never been through a depression, and when I was hurting the most, I needed him the most. *But I couldn't always explain what I needed.* Though we have now been together thirty-one years, he rarely knows what state I'm in. He's probably heard me talk about 3,000 different mood changes, and he still believes life will be OK.

Evan and I were married in 1979 and were very excited and in love. It was all hypomanic for me, since my lithium was not helping to stabilize me. Shortly after the wedding in Illinois, Evan took a job in California, which meant a huge move, from Colorado to California. The trip out there turned out to be an adventure I'd just as soon forget.

Manic episodes: An extremely elevated mood characterized by excessive energy, impulsivity, impaired judgement, irritability, a decreased need for sleep, and may be accompanied by paranoia and psychoses

One's destination
is never a place,
but a new way
of seeing things.

—Henry Miller

5 Cross Country Moves

M oving across state lines requires big changes, which are tough for me. Moves are difficult because it takes months to settle in, and I can't wait that long. Finding a new home, making new friends, and trying to get oriented are challenges in my unstable state.

The anxiety grows, as I imagine all the details of the move, and I become overwhelmed. Each day, as my husband discusses more projects we must do, I lose more touch with reality; but this doesn't show because I keep moving. It is always an "episode," but few people have ever observed me going through it. I hide it well.

1972 • Colorado

My first major move was from my hometown in Illinois to Colorado, where I attended the University of Denver. I drove out with my parents (no big deal) and made an almost immediate adjustment to friends and school. I was hypomanic for one year, so everything was easy. I was lucky because, if I had been even moderately depressed, I wouldn't have started college. I remember a big blur of fun, studies, and trips to the mountains. It was a rare year in my life to be hypomanic for such a long time with no worries.

> *Finding a new home, making new friends, and trying to get oriented are big challenges in my unstable state.*

But the hypomania wore off, and by my junior and senior years I gradually plunged into the familiar pattern of difficulty sleeping and concentrating, as well as depression. It was an irritable depression; my head felt tight and chaotic at the same time. I had no patience with myself or other people. I rarely relaxed. This was normal for me. Every day I felt confined to my brain; yet, I was tough enough to keep going. It was a familiar package I was able to handle, but it scared me to imagine my future in this state of mind.

1978 • California

When I met my husband, Evan, after I graduated from college, he was working in Denver. After we got married, he took another job in his field, and we moved from Denver to California. It was around this time that I was diagnosed as manic-depressive and started taking lithium. I knew my life was going to be better than before; I trusted the medication. I was overly excited about getting married and out of control, but I was fighting to remain calm by exercising and doing other positive things for myself.

My second move, from Colorado to Los Angeles, was in my grandfather's old Bel Air, which I believed I could drive cross-country. This ride was an episode, for sure. I recall being so determined to get to L.A. to see Evan, it didn't matter to me what trauma I had to go through to get there.

I probably needed more medication, but I was moving and not thinking about how I could change my manic behavior. I made a big mistake by driving by myself to L.A. I should have shipped my car there and flown to LAX, but I had no money. Some work friends at the nursing home made me a going-away gift box with all kinds of surprise snacks and gadgets for my trip. In the box was No-Doz, which I thought would keep me awake and alert. I just took them like candy; in my system, they were horrific. I was hyped up, jittery, and extremely nervous; at the same time, I felt as if I wasn't really there.

In addition, the exhaust system in my car was failing, and I had all the windows open because I had no air conditioning. I was breathing in fumes and getting intoxicated, just floating across the country unaware of my surroundings until I stopped for gas, with my muffler dragging under the car. The mechanic looked at me and said, "You are grounded, lady, for three hours. No driving!"

Once back on the road, I was sinking and feeling very sick by this time but compelled to keep going. The San Bernardino Mountains were beckoning, and I remember slowing the car down to fifteen miles per hour to see if I was still on the road. The sky was so blue, the sun was shining; but I was hanging on by a thread. It was the first hallucination I had created for myself, and it was terrifying. Arriving in L.A., I got lost and had to stop to ask someone if I could use the phone to call Evan. The people where I stopped said sure. They were all having a party and doing the strangest drugs. I was scared.

Evan couldn't locate me and also got lost. When he finally did pick me up, we drove another two or three hours to get to his place. It took me a full week to recover. I slept all day, then listened to disco music and drank Coca-Cola to try to wake up.

In California, I had a new batch of symptoms. I became depressed and very anxious. I started having physical problems—irritable colon and migraines—and I couldn't stop any of them. By that time I had a new job, but I felt frozen and unable to fit in. The job required a master's degree in science, which I didn't have, but I felt I had to keep working. I wanted to prove myself.

I remember rough edges and battling myself as I tried

to figure out why I was such a wreck. What I didn't know was that, every time a person with bipolar disorder has a new symptom, it seems like a brand-new situation. I was confused at first, but once I realized this, I was able to be more patient with myself. I kept taking one lithium a day to stabilize my moods, but I had no idea I could increase my dose or take an antidepressant as well. (I had already been depressed for most of ten years.) But, oh, did I enjoy walking the beach and finding sea creatures and eating seafood and traveling the countryside.

1982 • Ohio

Evan's job changed again, and so we began a new adventure in Ohio. I was in a very delicate state from my stay in California and would soon crash. We arrived in a snowstorm, which seemed to last forever. After the bitter cold, the dark clouds, along with a very sneaky depression, sapped most of my energy. I would say this depression lasted for three years, but I was also a bundle of anxiety. It was all mixed together. My husband was in a fine mood, but he kept trying to understand what seemed like a new condition for me. I was embarrassed by how much he did to help me. I was practically nonfunctioning in some ways. Then, I developed wild symptoms in my body and mind. The worst was nerve-ending pain that affected my body, fingers and toes, legs, arms, and head. This was another new condition that kicked me in the face because I couldn't understand it. Meanwhile, I was crying all day, refusing to get out of bed. The pain felt like little pinches or pricks and was very distracting. I'd never heard of anyone getting this, and I was horrified. For months, I took pain medicine, which accomplished nothing. Finally, I was admitted to the hospital, where I underwent tests for six days.

The nurses, I remember, didn't want to talk with me much. My neurologist, after ruling out all kinds of diseases, believed I needed a bit of Elavil for the nerve-ending pain. Since I looked depressed to him, he referred me to a psychiatrist at Ohio State University. I think this was the second time I did not get to a psychiatrist in time to help me.

The psychiatrist recommended that I take a bigger dose of Elavil; he expected results. After months of playing with the drug, the light cracked through my system, and I began enjoying life again! This was before Prozac, and Elavil had many rough edges. It was my first antidepressant, just one of many I would try in the years to come.

My psychiatrist was compassionate and knowledgeable about counseling and drug management. He was very rare. He could do talk therapy and manage medications at the same time. He also provided Evan and me with genetic counseling. At some point after that, psychiatry moved from a talking therapy to drug management only. I believe many suffer from the lack of human contact in a business that once treated patients with care and compassion.

My psychiatrist was compassionate and knowledge-able about counseling and drug management. He was very rare.

Throughout this whole ordeal, Evan would still listen to me, hoping for some recovery. I think he knew I would get better because he had been through plenty of ups and downs with me already. And, eventually, I did get better.

After being in an apartment for six months, we bought a house. The next phase of our move was to transport our furniture to our new house. Evan drove the truck and told me to ride in the back of the truck to stabilize the furniture. Unfortunately, a mirror broke during the ride, and I had several cuts and was bleeding. I became enraged; when we stopped at our house, I picked up our pieces of furniture and threw them down, breaking several of them. My strength was magnified; I was unaware of my body's power. My last memory was hurling a very heavy sewing machine, which also smashed to pieces on the street. I became my rage; strangely, it was a good feeling.

1984 • St. Louis

Our move to St. Louis was exhilarating, as I was confident and very energetic. My goal was, in only two weeks, to move and empty all our boxes, while landscaping in ninety-five-degree weather. I gradually became hypomanic and worked twelve to fourteen hours each day with few or no breaks. Evan was happy to see me tackling so many projects (ha!) and had no idea that my bipolar change would lead to my eventual crash. No clues could stop me from abusing my body.

But after three weeks of intense labor and feeling no pain, I developed pneumonia and was unable to continue. I slept several hours a day and was still exhausted. Through this experience, I learned the consequences of overworking my body while I was in a hypomanic state. Six weeks later, I was able to return to my projects. The move to St. Louis was still great because I was not depressed and remained in excellent spirits.

> *After several moves—at ages eighteen, twenty-five, and thirty-two—I have learned how to protect myself when I am making a move and how to prioritize the aspects of the move.*

Rather than remembering the frustration and anxiety associated with relocating, I recall the highlights of exploring new places. My husband and I loved new experiences in new locales. As long as we took risks, our lives became more fulfilling. After several moves—at ages eighteen, twenty-five, and thirty-two—I have learned how to protect myself when I am making a move and how to prioritize the aspects of the move. As I get older, I seem to handle moves better.

It's OFTEN thE
LɑST KEY ON thE riNq
thɑt OPENS thE door.

—Doris LESSINq

6 Medication Games

Medication is one of my favorite topics because it is the key to a bipolar sufferer's stability and well-being. Medications work, but they are complicated and need constant monitoring for symptoms and response. I have struggled to keep medications working with my unique chemical system. Everyone has a different system, but taking medications is like trying on new clothes. Sometimes, they don't fit; sometimes, they are the wrong color; sometimes, they make us look fat or too old or too conservative. Finally, we find the right outfit, but it takes time. We buy the clothes and wear them and hope they last. Sometimes, they don't.

There are people who don't accept taking medication. For them, medication is like a pollutant or unknown substance. Even if those of us with bipolar are hesitant to put anything foreign in our bodies, we still have major problems like depression and mania to solve. Ultimately, we must put our faith in medications with good track records that will work in our systems to balance us and make it possible to live healthy lives.

Medications work, but they are complicated and need constant monitoring for symptoms and response.

From age twelve, I had bipolar disorder, but lithium had not yet been widely accepted for use in psychiatry. So I jumped from depression to hypomania, wishing someone or something would stop my craziness. I gave ten or more psychiatrists and therapists plenty of time to help me find my way, but I always ended up in the same place. I even began to accept myself as doomed. When I began taking lithium in the seventies, I knew I was going in the right direction. I had spent too much time in pain and essentially untreated; my new drug was my salvation.

New Drug Regimen

I had just started taking a new drug, one of the best new antidepressants on the market. I was excited. I was always thinking about improving my life. The goal was for me to be less sedated and have more energy. This had been going on for five years. I was always taking naps, and it made me feel lazy. I was prescribed Lexapro, which had an immediate effect on me. I began moving around and doing a lot. Wow! It felt like being on amphetamines. The question was, would it last? It felt as if my mind was being controlled, but then everything became agitated in my brain—not good.

Occasionally, I would wake at night and for two hours I would clean, decorate, file, and organize. This was too good to be true; I'm never that efficient. One day I had the most perfect day: Everything was clear, I had energy, I had no anxiety, and I could have sailed if I had a boat. These kinds of days happened, but *how* did they happen?

However, my intolerance for the agitation was such that I had to discontinue Lexapro. It took a full three weeks before I realized I'd have to go off it. This medicine was too powerful for me. I experienced good things with the drug, but they were outweighed by the bad.

What I have learned is that I will not tolerate a feeling of agitation. It feels as if there is some rotted matter in my brain, or pieces of metal, or extra lines moving in a direction so that I can actually feel extra movement. At other times, I want to scream or smash my head on the wall to get some of the agitation out. Not many people would understand what I am talking about, and the rest would not want to. But I think that when we have funny or unusual feelings in our brains, we need to contact our doctors as soon as possible.

Time Frame

It usually takes one to four weeks for a drug to work. It is difficult to be patient at this time because I wonder about the outcome. Will the drug work? Sometimes, the chemicals are not in balance until the drug is performing well, and sometimes I feel agitation. In some cases with an antidepressant, I actually feel more depression, temporarily, until the drug kicks in. When that happens, I definitely need counseling from my doctor because I am feeling insecure and anxious. A couple of words from the doctor can really help me to endure until the next medical appointment.

Going Off a Drug

Going off a drug is a special circumstance. Usually, the drug is decreased so gradually that I can't even tell the medication has been deleted from my system. Occasionally, stopping a drug may cause withdrawal, which is an unlovely experience—a total mind-body reaction that includes vision problems, nausea, headaches, irritability, and panicky feelings. My skin feels as if it's crawling inside my head. I can't fight a withdrawal, but I certainly let someone know about it. I like to be walked through the experience day by day with kind, supportive words.

Substituting One Drug for Another

When one drug is omitted and another one substituted in

its place, the plan is to proceed slowly. The doctor calcu-
lates the timing so that there is definite overlap between
both drugs.

> *Taking new drugs, juggling the drugs, being patient,*
> *and acting assertive with the medical profession are*
> *ways to cope with this overpowering disorder.*

One time, when a new medication was replacing an old
one, my overly sensitive system missed the connection
between my two drugs; I became severely depressed
within three days, so that I couldn't eat or drink anything.
I could not even manage to raise myself out of bed. Every
day, I would try to drink Ensure and attempt to sit up.
It was a horrible, unreal situation; I felt I was moving
toward nonexistence. My family kept encouraging me and
cooking for me, but I was a basket case. I was frightened
and completely nonfunctional. I kept up the communication with the doctor. I knew my replacement drug was
being increased each day, and, after an agonizing week,
I got up and started living again. It was a very strange
occurrence. It made me realize that I would never be able
to go without an antidepressant. Ever.

My Symbiotic Relationship with Lithium
Lithium, one of the best bipolar mood stabilizers, was my
main staple for thirty years. But at age fifty-three, hand

tremors caused by lithium were a big problem that affected my computer use, writing, drawing, piano playing, and eating. Often in the morning, I had to hold the orange juice glass with two hands. My psychiatrist and I thought I could try a new mood stabilizer, although it would be a risk. Generally, I had to feel strong and confident before I engaged in a big project like changing medications. I dropped my lithium for the first time and began the new medication. I could tell it wasn't working, but I knew that I had to reach a high dose before the actual change would begin.

At first, I became hypomanic with bursts of energy, which I used by working in my garden and house and writing. Each day became more intense. I would have stopped moving around so much, but my mind and body were racing out of control. I was completely self-centered and was barely aware of anyone else. For three months, my life rambled into mania. This was a scary time for me.

Soon my mind was racing so fast, I couldn't focus on any tasks, and there seemed no reason to exist. I had lost it, and others were noticing. Lights flashed when I was driving, and I became lost several times but luckily returned home to safety. I got a piece of paper and wrote down the things I had to do at the bottom of the page. I carried the sheet with me during the day so I knew what I should focus on. I could finish something if my mind was glued to the paper; otherwise, I couldn't.

Without lithium, I dropped into a deep depression for short periods; then, the rest of the day I was manic. I felt fragile. Was this how I would always be without a mood stabilizer? Maybe this was why I was maintained on lithium for so long. My body and muscles were included in this manic episode. For four days, I worked on home projects, taxing my knees, lifting, and pushing. By the fifth day, my entire body was stiff and aching. With some medication and much rest, in six weeks I was finally able to go on my usual walk. This overuse syndrome caused by my mania had occurred a few other times in my life. When I am working fast, I do not feel pain and cannot stop myself. I pay for it later with physical therapy.

Just as I had gone off lithium, I went back on lithium. I was comfortable, able to use my brain again and to start living a reasonable life. My psychiatrist said that lithium was my drug, and I knew this was the truth.

Drug History Chart

It is difficult to keep track of medications and dosages, especially if there have been many of them over the years. As new doctors tried to find the best drug or combination of drugs to treat my condition, I have kept a record of what I was taking. That way, if a new medication, or what seemed like a new medication, was prescribed, I could look at my record to determine if I had taken it in the past. Over time, I developed a drug history chart that includes the drug name, dosage, effectiveness, side effects, and start and end dates for every medication. Keeping track of my medications from the time of my diagnosis has already saved time and prevented confusion and will continue to do so in the future.

I have included a sample chart on the next page.

Sample Drug History Chart

Drug	Positive Effects/Symptoms	Negative Effects/Symptoms	Start Date	End Date

The underlying current of
family support is what created
self-confidence for me.

The good part is that
family is forever.

— Marti Markley

7 Family Ties

Like anyone who has a chronic, major disease, a person with bipolar disorder needs support, especially from family. If parents, siblings, or significant others are not available, occasionally grandparents, aunts, uncles, cousins, or friends can meet this need. If there are no family or friends participating, an organized support group (typically at a hospital) is often a good way to talk about problems with medications, symptoms, jobs, and other life issues.

The most important thing a family can do is become educated about the disease, its symptoms, and what to expect. Empathy is a crucial component of helping people with bipolar disorder achieve comfort, even when their progress is slow. Unfortunately, some people simply do not make supportive caregivers. They don't understand that chemicals cause depression and mood swings, and they

seem to expect their sick relative to motivate and eventually cure himself or herself. Friends or family may even try
to suggest that the person with bipolar discontinue taking
medications because of their own unwarranted distrust
and dislike of medicines.

*The most important thing a family can do is become
educated about the disorder, its symptoms, and
what to expect.*

Somewhere at the beginning of the diagnosis period,
a person with bipolar disorder will have to cope with
the stigma of the disease. It is a long road from there to
understanding bipolar and developing a strong sense of
self. There are so many questions: Am I comfortable with
my own diagnosis? Who should know about my illness?
Will it be beneficial or harmful to tell friends, people at
work, others? What boundaries would I like to keep? What
privacy issues are important to me?

There are several programs that work to reduce the
stigma associated with mental illness. According to Jan
Fawcett, MD, author of *New Hope for People with Bipolar
Disorder*, one such program funded by the New Alliance for
Mental Illness (NAMI) advocates compassion and educa-
tion. Another, sponsored by the American Psychological
Association (APA) and the Depressive and Manic-Depres-
sive Association (DMDA), uses hotlines and brochures to

get information to teenagers and young adults. There is a plethora of information out there to help people with bipolar disorder become knowledgeable and comfortable with current therapeutic trends. We need to learn everything we can about our own illness through books, memoirs, workshops, support groups, and the Internet.

Parents and Siblings

Because I was only twelve when my condition became apparent for the first time, I was living at home with my parents, who were my main source of support. They were shocked at all my symptoms, but they listened to me and approved of the therapy sessions I was attending twice a week at the state hospital. They kept me moving with my schoolwork and friendships, which was a great tactic. We did not understand my disease, and that was frustrating. The diagnosis didn't come until eleven years later. My parents were there for me. I knew it; so, I kept going, hoping to find a way out of my misery. My brothers and sisters seemed to be curious, but they did not get involved in my drama. I accepted this as the way it was.

After I left home at eighteen, I didn't feel like telling everyone my story and don't even recall knowing anyone with depression or bipolar disorder. I was isolated, but I had gotten used to that. When I met my husband, he was very supportive, but since we moved often, I could not rely on a set group of friends for support. In addition, my family was never available to me. They all live up north, at least ten hours away. I would like to be around my parents, my three brothers and sister, my aunts and uncles and forty cousins; but it will never happen. On the other hand, my small dog, Chupa, is 100 percent in my corner no matter what I do. She gives me love that keeps my heart feeling warm. A pet is a great thing to have under any circumstances, but especially when one is battling a chronic illness.

Heredity and Bipolar Disorder

Bipolar disorder is a genetic vulnerability that runs in families. My younger brother had his first episode when he was seventeen, but it was mania, not depression. We are seven years apart, and he lives many miles away; yet we function almost like bipolar twins. After his diagnosis, we realized the importance of staying in touch, and we have developed our own two-person support group by telephone. We are keen to find out the new information on medications and therapies, and we keep each other informed. As similar as our heredity is, though, we do not take any of the same medications.

Regardless of where my particular "genetic vulnerability" came from, I wanted to know whether my bipolar genes would transfer to my children. What was the probability of having a son or daughter with bipolar? I could just imagine a wonderful child, normal, with no mood disorders, depressions, or mania. On the other hand, I could also imagine my child with a full-blown mania or depression. It was not a pretty picture.

My psychiatrist told me that the odds were possibly one in three that my children might be manic-depressive. I didn't like the odds. If there is a possibility of passing on this disease, family planning is extremely important. He suggested that we have one biological child and adopt another. As years passed, I realized I had followed his formula, although I never planned to. (I have two children, nine years apart—one biological and one adopted.)

My psychiatrist told me that the odds were possibly one in three that my children might be manic-depressive. I didn't like the odds.

Delicate Choices
Choice 1: Getting pregnant
After three years of marriage, Evan and I were ready to plan a pregnancy. I knew this would be a difficult project because, at the time, I had major depression and only two menstrual periods a year. Tests indicated I was normal, but my gynecologist was skeptical and told me I didn't have a good chance of getting pregnant. I was taking lithium and an antidepressant. I began by going off medications for two months so there would be no toxicity in my body; and I followed all doctor's orders.

In addition, I took my stress and stomped it into the ground. I quit my job and started landscaping our home. I was experimenting, but I knew that to be depressed and highly anxious would not work. Gradually, my periods came back, though there seemed to be no real reason for that change. And like a bolt of lightning, I became pregnant with my first and only daughter. No one believed me when I told them my happy news, not even my father.

As she grew up, my daughter seemed to develop a personality like my husband's. She was not in a rush, she had a pleasing way about her, and she was a bit shy. As she grew older, I would point out to my husband the differences between our daughter and me. We would say, "Yes, we beat the bipolar game." We were lucky.

Choice 2: Having an abortion

One year later, a fiasco occurred that sent me into mass confusion and grief. I became pregnant while taking medications. Most people would have the baby and be happy, but I did not have a choice to have a baby because lithium causes defects in the heart in the first month of development. Even though I was just a few days pregnant, damage was happening. There was no time for treatments (there were none, anyway); I had to think fast and be clear about my decision. Each day was torture because I was trapped. I could not be a part of creating a baby who would suffer, even though I wanted this baby. My doctors told me my best option was to have an abortion, and that's what I did.

Nine months later I got pregnant again, while taking all my medications and using birth control—the Today sponge. I was angry because the birth control was supposed to work, but I had no time to contact the company and voice my strong opinion. Again, I did my own research in medical books and asked gynecologists whether I had any options. Again, the doctors advised an abortion—my second. I knew I was being responsible, but I was again devastated.

Choice 3: Tubal ligation

After my experiences with unintended pregnancies, I decided to have a tubal ligation. I wasn't having any more children. I was happy with only one child, so the tubal ligation would provide me with a great sense of relief. I believe people with bipolar disorder find life easier and less stressful with fewer children. It is difficult to manage manic-depression while taking care of a household, a job, and children at the same time. The tubal ligation was a very final and scary decision, but I have never regretted it.

Choice 4: Adopting a child

My daughter was doing well at nine. I was stable, and I thought about how much time I had for another child.

Evan and I looked into an international adoption. Within a year, we had a wonderful eighteen-month-old Filipino son.

When Bipolar Affects Children

Each child reacts differently to a parent with bipolar disorder. Sometimes, it is difficult to tell how the children are reacting, so it might be a good idea to get third-party input. It is the parent's "sickness" that can worry children. Do they comprehend what bipolar is, or do they compare it to the flu or stomach problems or migraines?

What if your mom lies around all day and doesn't have energy like she "used to"? What if she doesn't talk much anymore or has lost her sense of humor? What if Mom is yelling and snapping at everyone, and she was never like that before? What if her facial expressions are different? Children are great observers and listeners and will notice every change in their parents' behavior. But can they understand a disease as complex as bipolar disorder? Probably not, because it takes several years for the person with bipolar to understand her own symptoms, fluctuations in behavior, and mood swings. How can a child be expected to grasp it?

My daughter avoided my bipolar disease from early childhood through her teenage years. Whenever I tried to discuss a problem, she ignored me! She didn't want to be a part of anything negative or any "sickness." She always enjoyed my energetic behavior, but she couldn't cope with my depressive side. I think my decline made her feel panicky and slightly irritated. I let her continue to deny my disease because I really didn't want her to know the depth of my pain, and I didn't want her to take responsibility for me.

I tried to keep up with all of her school and social activities even though it was hard to focus and be energetic at times. I felt satisfied and content when I knew her needs had been met. During difficult times, I felt inadequate, even though I was trying. I wanted a "normal" life for my kids.

My son knew that something was wrong with me from the time he was seven. He would come up to me when I was lying down and want to know if I was sick or had a headache, or "what." He seemed worried. I wished I didn't feel crummy or depressed or need to crash on the couch. I guess he preferred that I not lie down at all. Later, when he was nine, he asked what bipolar was, and I explained it to him. He had overheard my husband and me talk about the changes I go through. Of course, a child does not understand this disease from listening to his parents, so it was a good move on my part to try to explain bipolar in a way that he could grasp.

Since bipolar disorder or manic-depression is not a common word or idea, parents have to explain it in simple terms to children. Children need to be reassured. They need to know that Mom is OK or *will be* OK and that the medications are helping her feel better. That knowledge keeps them from guessing about what's wrong. Children may wonder if theirs is the only parent with bipolar. After all, I did not meet another person with this condition until I was thirty years old; that was after *eighteen* years of living in isolation with this disease.

Since bipolar disorder or manic-depression is not a common word or idea, parents have to explain it in simple terms to children. Children need to be reassured.

National Association for Mental Illness (NAMI): A grassroots mental health advocacy organization dedicated to improving the lives of individuals and families affected by mental illness

If he could get inside my head

And make sense of my evasive moods,

It would help both of us convey
our thoughts and feelings more
clearly.

— Marti Markley

8 My Husband's Perspective

I was initially attracted to Marti because of her free-spir-
ited, lively, and somewhat zany personality. She was
an intense, artistic person. In 1977, when we began
our relationship, we were twenty-four. Marti gradually
told me about her very new diagnosis of bipolar disorder.
I was unaware of this condition. She talked about turmoil
in her head. I listened, but I didn't think it would affect her
in any great way. A year after we were married, I was still
not at all concerned about her mental health. I saw my
wife as lively and very capable. At that time, her energy
was perhaps a disguise, a hypomanic mode she was experiencing but unaware of.

Within the first two years, I had witnessed both her
depression and mania. When she was manic, she talked
and moved quickly and didn't sleep well. She was taking a
small amount of lithium, which helped somewhat. I wasn't

involved in her psychiatric treatment or medications. We did go to some support group events, but I felt she was in control of her overall health. In reality, her moods were not stabilized, and I did not understand them. We were happy and had few problems. I believe she knew there were rough times ahead, as they had continued since she was twelve, but it was unimaginable to view my wife as mentally ill.

I remember one manic episode at the ocean when she dove into the water, wrapped herself in seaweed, and came out laughing and jumping up and down. These were actually happy times for me—events that were fun. There were many other times when she was overly excited, but I found her entertaining. These times stick in my mind more firmly than the down swings.

I believe she knew there were rough times ahead, as they had continued since she was twelve, but it was unimaginable to view my wife as mentally ill.

I have seen Marti go through about four depressions, and these were baffling times for me. Although she was taking medication, the depression took over her mind and body, lasted many months, and ranged from moderate to severe. I was learning that living with a person with bipolar caused our family extra chaos, and I couldn't fix it. I did not make it a major project to research the disorder, and I'm not sure why. After ten years of living together, the good in our marriage still outweighed the bad.

Once, after our move from California to Ohio, Marti became very depressed. She took painkillers the doctor prescribed but stayed at home in our new, unappealing apartment. I had a new job, so I only saw her after work. She was unable to cope, and I remember feeling very helpless, especially since she was stubborn and wouldn't listen to my suggestions. She was giving in to her disease, and I was watching her do it. I always had a great deal of hope. It helped to have seen her in her good times, which proved to me that we would get out of the hole, eventually. I am a calm person and don't worry much, a trait that has helped our relationship.

The preparation to have kids required a lot of planning. The lithium had to be stopped in order to conceive a healthy baby. Our first child was born healthy and without medications. Unfortunately, Marti got pregnant twice after our daughter was born and had two abortions, which were recommended by all her doctors. Those were traumatic situations. Eventually, we adopted a child from the Philippines.

The preparation to have kids required a lot of planning. The lithium had to be stopped in order to conceive a healthy baby.

The family now tries to manage around Marti's compromised life. We feel sympathetic about her bipolar symptoms, though our lives are not terribly diminished. Marti, however, misses out on many activities when she can't cope, takes time-outs, or needs to slow down. Loss of energy and lethargy are probably her main symptoms that have affected our children. When I could see that she was going through a low time, I took over some of her responsibilities, like driving the kids to their activities, grocery shopping, and doing extra housework.

The children seemed to accept that sometimes she had to take naps, but she was always there for them when they came home from school. Our family is more energized when Marti is up, humorous, outgoing, and even hypomanic. That's when she creates art, plays music, and dances, all activities she engages in that unify our family.

For many years, frequent migraines interfered with her stability. Migraines hit in a random pattern, so fixing them is very difficult. She has changed her life to accommodate lost time on these days, and I know she has been forced to do so. There are no options here. I would like to think these down times are positively offset by the good times we often share.

Because my wife is sometimes hypomanic, our communications can be difficult. She is usually thinking one to three thoughts ahead of our conversation, and I occasionally lose track of what we are talking about. In addition, Marti talks in a reverse sequence pattern and tells me the topic *after* she has described the details, or she begins with the conclusion and *then* introduces the topic. This has gone on for thirty years and is very frustrating. Her free-floating way of talking makes me have to stop and figure out what she is really saying.

Marti is quick to move. She frequently jumps up when she is ready to go to the car or the store or leave a restaurant, and she doesn't stay with our family group. Her impulsive behavior sometimes annoys me. Of course, she leaves her keys, purse, or coat behind, even when she's medicated. I believe she is highly distracted and can't focus on one task at a time. However, she has accomplished much in her life, and maybe I take her successes for granted.

Adjusting to new places, whether a new home, a vacation, or a weekend trip, has always been very difficult for her. We would often have to change plans and split up because Marti needed extra time to reduce her stress level. She might stay in the hotel or go for a walk to try to relax and figure out why her chemicals had switched. I, on the other hand, am very physically active and want to be outside exploring my new environment. After a few days, life becomes more enjoyable again. I am always encouraging Marti to continue physical activity, but I know it's difficult for her or anyone to stick to a good program.

Both the depressive and hypomanic poles create irritability in my wife, which was an issue because I would feel sensitive to her comments. She kept saying, "Why can't you see that I am having a difficult time and give me a break?" But once again, I could not read her bipolar symptoms, so we became irritated with each other.

Identifying triggers that could exacerbate her bipolar symptoms was a gradual learning process for me. Triggers are really environmental factors. They can't be eliminated, but I can make small changes to prevent intense behavior on her part. Knowing what these triggers are can save time and prevent mood outbreaks, according to Julie A. Fast in *Loving Someone with Bipolar Disorder* (New Harbinger Publications, Inc. 2004). I can anticipate that traveling will be a trigger, as will lack of exercise, too many obligations, being constantly on the move, and over-scheduling activities. These triggers are predictable.

Identifying triggers that could exacerbate her bipolar symptoms was a gradual learning process for me.

Marti's support group consists of a large number of doctors, her parents, her brother, her close friends, and our immediate family. Both of our families live out of state, so we are unable to rely on them for support when difficult times arise. But we also have a simpler life and do less entertaining over the holidays. As a result, we have less stress and fewer obligations. We still want to see our relatives more often than we are able to. This family situation is a trade-off because we can't be included in many of the family dinners and parties.

Getting the correct meds is critical. For Marti these seem to be a cocktail of lithium and other drugs that needs constant monitoring to stabilize her condition, which is often cycling. One of my strategies to make myself feel as if I am sorting out the chaos of Marti's life is to get her to list all her medications, periodically, and to ask her whether these medications are working. But when the medications are changed, I often become confused. I thought I could match her symptoms with her medications and be helpful in this way, but this has not proved to be a beneficial strategy because of the complex and constantly changing nature of bipolar.

Another strategy I have learned over the years is to ask Marti what her next move would be, in specific terms, when she is having problems. One example is to ask her if she needs to make another appointment with her psychiatrist, or go for a walk, or cancel any obligations for the next day to make life easier. These are suggestions on my part that seem to be effective.

We know that, as changes occur in her life with bipolar, we will be making small changes maybe monthly, weekly, or daily. Marti may go through a variety of frustrating times, and I still can't understand all the dimensions of the bipolar disorder. But I will continue to be her number one support person. I also believe that, as a couple, we have lasted in a bipolar relationship for a long time, and that is a rewarding accomplishment.

Trigger: Something external that can set in motion an oncoming bipolar episode; can be caused by stress, a major disappointment, or something as simple as a poor night's sleep

Traveling is a brutality.

It forces you to trust strangers and lose sight of all that familiar comfort of home and friends.

You are constantly out of balance.

Nothing is yours except the essential things — air, sleep, dreams, the sea, the sky — all things tending towards the eternal or what we imagine.

— Cesare Pavese

9 Vacations

Vacations are supposed to be relaxing and fun—enjoyable times spent with the family. To me, vacations can be times of insurmountable stress. A week before I leave, my excitement begins to build, and I cannot stop it. Typically, I am overexcited and my brain feels numb, almost like being depressed. I don't sleep well. My excitement level increases every hour prior to traveling. My head feels tight, so I do all kinds of relaxation techniques and go for walks in the wilderness. But I still carry around this head full of the wrong kind of jazz. My doctors have encouraged me to exercise every day before I leave, take more medication, and keep taking it until I begin to relax. Sometimes it works after four days; sometimes it may take up to a week; sometimes it doesn't work at all.

When I am depressed, the trip seems difficult. But, because I want to travel and experience new events, I rely more on people and take fewer risks. When I'm overexcited, I get anxious. Over the years I've tried new amounts of medication before I leave on my trip and new techniques while I am vacationing. I have learned many ways to stop this wild pattern, but I always have to plan before I travel. Usually, I have difficulties on one or two out of three trips; but, within the last twenty years, I have improved! I am getting better at juggling all the excitement.

My doctors have encouraged me to exercise every day before I leave, take more medication, and keep taking it until I begin to relax.

My goal when I am away is to keep experiencing the fun of a vacation with my family, even though I may feel off. I am aware of my surroundings and enjoy new activities, whether I am overexcited or not. I am patient with myself and wait for a change to occur in my head. After the daily activities, I take two hours to unwind, read, or do something by myself. If I can avoid gastrointestinal problems or migraines, I am doing well.

No one in my circle of family or friends is a handicapped traveler. They do not have drastic changes to cope with. Often, I don't sleep well while I'm away. When I arrive home, I need three or four days to recover from the excitement. I feel as if I am upside down. I try not to schedule any appointments on these recovery days.

*No one in my circle of family or friends is a handi-
capped traveler. They do not have drastic changes
to cope with.*

Occasionally, however, I do manage to ease myself into
the vacation with stability and no distressing symptoms.
Wow, I feel so human when I can enjoy a holiday the way
other people do! Despite all that, I am always glad I had the
opportunity to go on a vacation and survive the experience.

Memorable Vacations
1969 • Age 15
I took the train from Illinois to Denver to go to a hiking and
horseback riding camp in Colorado. Even though I was
depressed, my psychologist and parents thought I might
enjoy a new environment. While I was there, though, I
was withdrawn, anxious, and reluctant to take risks. Life
was very confusing, and I was afraid. The camp lasted
a month, but my depression stayed with me after it was
over. The high altitude was great, though, and my senses
did allow me to take in the gorgeous mountains. It was
probably the best place I have ever been.

1970 • Age 16
My family and I were vacationing at a small hotel. The
weather was hot, so we all went to check out the small
swimming pool. For three weeks, I had been very

depressed and fearful, unmotivated, unhappy, dark, and gloomy. I had been through two years of changes from depression to hypomania, and I never knew when they would occur. I lowered myself into the water, and suddenly my eyes were flooded with iridescent greens and blues, hot light crashing at every angle. Within two minutes, I had a breakthrough into a manic state, and I screamed for joy. I thrashed in the water, intensely aware that I had left my depression behind. My chemicals had created a nice miracle for me and given me precious time to feel superb.

I feel so human when I can enjoy a holiday the way other people do. I am always glad I had the opportunity to go on a vacation and survive the experience.

1982 • Age 28

I flew to Florida to visit my parents. I was OK when I left, but then I discovered I had left all my medications at home. I very quickly went into a withdrawal and had a bad headache, so I stayed in bed. I was irritable, and my stomach was queasy. We telephoned home and had my medications mailed, but I was out of commission for twenty-four hours. Everyone seemed bummed out. Within twelve hours of getting back on my medications, I was feeling good, relaxed, and even. The rest of the trip was fine. To this day, my husband questions me several times

before we leave for a trip—"Do you have your medications?"—and I have to show them to him.

1990 • Age 36

While boarding a plane, I experienced an instantaneous
mental and physical collapse. I was headed to California
with Evan, who was attending a workshop for four days.
It was supposed to be a relaxing and enjoyable time for
me. Initially, on the plane I became hysterical, and I knew
something was very wrong. Was one of my medications
causing this, or was my head changing? I couldn't figure
it out. And I couldn't fix it. I lost my appetite, sleep was
scarce, and it was alarming that I couldn't sit or stand.
Sightseeing was out of the question, and I lay in bed for
four days. I forgot, somehow, that I could call my psychiatrist. The last night we went out to dinner, and I lay down
in the restaurant booth, unable to sit up. When I returned
home, my doctors were confused by my symptoms and
suggested I go into the hospital, but this was only one
option for me. I begged them to change my medications,
and they agreed to do so.

1996 • Age 42

I drove to Minnesota with my family. I exercised for three
days before I left and took more mood stabilizers each
day. Luck was with me, and I was not overexcited the
entire trip. In fact, I was relaxed, confident, and satisfied.

2003 • Age 49

I traveled to Connecticut to visit my daughter at her house and to vacation on Martha's Vineyard. I was keyed up when I left but doing well when I arrived. Then, I became unglued and had colon and headache problems. I kept doing things because I desperately wanted to see the sights, but I had to take naps, hoping they would make me stronger. I had a few panicky periods, which was unusual for me. I got very nauseated and couldn't eat. I didn't want my daughter to think I was pathetic. At least she had not inherited my disorder. My daughter was relaxed and comfortable as she showed me around. I had no idea how I got in that mental or physical state.

2006 – 2007 • Age 49

Between 2006 and 2008, we traveled as a family to California and Arizona. I spent the time feeling uptight and wondered why I even bothered traveling at all. Certainly, no one said I had to. Occasionally, I was overwhelmed; but sometimes the vacation was fun, and I was amazed at the great beauty. Maybe when I get old, I will stay home and watch the travel channel on TV. It's bound to be less stressful.

2008 • Age 54

I was excited to take a trip to Minnesota to visit my family for a mega party of ninety Irish relatives. In the car, I couldn't concentrate. I didn't relax the entire trip. I tried exercising, taking daily walks, but these tricks did nothing to alleviate my pain. I continued to fight the mania any way I could. I was not successful.

2009 • Age 55

Likewise, on my trip to Ohio, I was miserable. I remember that no one seemed aware of my mania. Everyone treated me kindly, even though my mind was racing, and I had trouble sleeping. I juggled my medications as much as I could, but it just wasn't working.

As the years went by, I became better able to predict what might trigger a manic episode and change my schedule rapidly to prevent one from occurring. After a while, vacations ceased to cause me so much anguish, and I was often able to enjoy myself.

HOPE is LiKE the SUN,
which as we journey toward it,
casts the shadow of our
burden behind us.

— S. SMiLES

easonal affective disorder (SAD), which is often associated with depression, is caused by a lack of sunshine
and a change in the biological clock. Symptoms include
sluggishness, irritability, increased appetite for pastries,
and oversleeping. Winter months without sunlight are the
hardest to cope with, but help is available in the form of
full-spectrum light that mimics the sun. Even one hour per
day of use can be very helpful. Full-spectrum light sources
include table lamps, light boxes, or visors. They can easily
be purchased online.

Dark and suffocating clouds lasting only a few days are
all it takes to make me depressed. It is an extra depression, different from my usual one. It is a real phenomenon
for people who need more sunshine throughout the fall
and winter months. The gray weather seeps into my eyes,
and, very quickly, I go down—not all the way, but enough

notches to feel an extra irritating depression take hold, firmly. I am always afraid at this time each year. It feels like a takeover, sort of like a kidnapping of my mind.

Dark and suffocating clouds lasting only a few days are all it takes to make me depressed. It is an extra depression, different from my usual one.

When I was a child, my mother tried to change the weather for me. She would say, "Oh, see, there is a little spot of sunshine in those clouds, and I think this afternoon it will be getting nice." I was hypersensitive to the weather, so she hoped for sunshine. Otherwise, I would be in a bad mood. The difficult part is separating the SAD depressions from the standard bipolar depression. Ways I combat the clouds include seeking a medication change; exercising outside, particularly when there are a few sunrays; and using light therapy.

I have a brother who can work outside in cold, cloudy, rainy, and snowy weather and remain cheerful and unaware of his surroundings. I watch him and think he must be a freak. But people with SAD have to find the sunrays; it's like a part-time job.

I talk about SAD to my friends, and they are interested because many of them feel the same way about the sunshine. They wonder how scientific the process and the treatment are. The medical psychiatric community accepts it as a real condition.

As a child, I did not know I was reacting to dark weather, but this reaction continued into adulthood. Even then, if I saw the crack of sun through my bedroom window, it charged me. The day would be bright; my actions would be strong.

People with SAD have to find the sunrays; it's like a part-time job.

Grey Clouds White Clouds

Grey clouds

They come in fall.
The brain is filled with grey masses.
The shapes of grey clouds are evil
And grey clouds offer a lack of light
Days go by with grey clouds.
Soon you feel cheated.
And then you become choked with grey clouds
Another life condition you can't cope with
Knowing sunshine is possible does not change
The dread you feel inside your head.

White clouds

I awake and soon feel the weight lifted.
Look. The sun has escaped from the grey masses
and is now a force.
I must have it.
Sun, hit my eyeballs, penetrate.
The white clouds, developing creations in the sky,
signify the coexistence of
Sun.
My brain is light, so glad I am.

— Marti Markley

Seasonal Affective Disorder (SAD): Also known as winter depression or winter blues, is a mood disorder in which people who have normal mental health throughout most of the year experience depressive symptoms in the winter year after year

To exist is to change,
to change is to mature,
to mature is to go on
creating oneself endlessly.

— Anonymous

11 ChaNgES

By definition, people with bipolar disorder experience many changes within our own physical and mental systems. The conditions in the brain are constantly changing, which causes chaos in our lives in the form of continually cycling mania and depression. However, many people have remissions and good months, even years. These are welcome changes.

The conditions in the brain are constantly changing, which causes chaos in our lives in the form of continually cycling mania and depression.

When we are stable, we want to work, volunteer, socialize, join groups, become productive members of society, discover our talents, and integrate with our families. All these activities bring about positive changes, but they are difficult to attain. Even when it is positive, the transitional process can be challenging.

Medication

Medications can produce major changes in the lives of people with bipolar. Sometimes, it takes a long time—possibly weeks—for the drugs to stabilize in the body. If one drug doesn't work, another one must be tried. Drugs, which cause side effects, have to be adjusted throughout a person's life. All these changes require patience and courage. The changes may be beneficial if the person with bipolar perseveres in the initial stage. A high percentage of people do achieve lasting and favorable results.

> *Sometimes, it takes a long time—possibly weeks—for the drugs to stabilize in the body.*

Notes on Life with Depression

- Lethargic, passive, no energy to get out of bed. The body has been poisoned by the mind. This is the last straw.

- Feeling sad and worthless and having difficulty doing ordinary jobs. I feel numb and unable to focus; concentration has left me.

- Now, things have changed drastically; life once again seems difficult, and my old pattern has taken hold.

- Is it possible that I have a fixed mechanism in my brain, like a button that is set for a certain period during which depression stagnates?

- Haven't been in this rotten of a mood in a long time—agitated—wanting to throw stones and yell and scream at everyone, but also wanting to cry. On the verge of something.

- I'm pulling through a thick mass. This is my life.

- There is a hole in my life. I feel deeply alone, but I can't fix it. It is a desperate feeling. Something has been taken from me.

- The agitation from depression takes over my brain, and I can feel a small area of my brain moving. I am edgy, but sometimes my doctor can fix it. Otherwise, it eats away at my brain. I can see it moving back and forth, and I would like to get rid of it. It is agitated depression.

- My sleep is always disturbed when I'm depressed. Maybe I've slept, but I feel tired. Usually, I awake several times during the night, but I always wake up early in the morning with great anxiety. I am fearful of my entire life, and I can't think myself out of it. The fear and anxiety come first, and then I begin thinking, Why? What will happen? What should I do? As I get up and join the living, my anxiety wanes.

- My head is in a black tunnel. I look and see the shadows of darkness everywhere and realize I have adjusted to this.

- When people look at me, I pretend to be normal. I don't want to talk, but I will give short answers that make sense so that no one knows I am depressed. I am trying to stay a part of this world, even though I am in left field. Instinctively, *I* need to protect myself.

Notes on Life with Hypomania/Mania

- Racing, talking fast, can't sit in a chair. Feel healthy and good. People at work think I am motivated. My head feels clear, devoid of depression; this hypomania can work for me.

- Sleeping is rough, like I am knocking myself against a wall.

- Agitation with a tendency to scream at people, think fast, and expect people to communicate instantly and be right. I feel edgy, and life is moving faster.

- I talk and move quickly. I'm filled with ideas and cross with people who get in my way. I attempt to overload myself with activities, which is only a temporary situation because I can't take the stress. Then, I have to cut back.

- I have tried so many ways to kill my insomnia. One method: No matter how awake I am, thinking a million thoughts, I will think every thought through until it is finished.

- No one questions my hypomania. People don't know I'm bipolar, as I project my camouflage.

- I am intuitively aware of people and their feelings.

- Laughing, not able to stop laughing, joking at parties, dancing up and down the halls with great physical intensity.

- Disco dancing, physically out of control but mentally planning my instant choreography, while paying homage to the heavy beat.

- I am optimistic, light, and forceful.

- Music makes me rise to the top of the world.

- In my head, I am chaotic, and life is moving fast.
  I am also very sensitive and touched by sad events.

Taking Charge of Change

My life has been all about change, beginning at age twelve, with psychiatrists, medications, and therapy. Cross-country moves and vacations were other changes I struggled with. At every turn I made, unforeseen bipolar variations drove me to distraction. However, I am accustomed to changes, and I rely on my strength to live one day at a time, to outwit both depression and mania. After forty years, I am changing the disorder as I once knew it. I have reached a place of power in my life.

My life has been all about change, beginning at age twelve, with psychiatrists, medications, and therapy.

EpiLOgUE

I n my fifties I developed a full-blown mixed mania, which was new to me and uncontrollable. My symptoms included distractibility, sleep problems, racing thoughts, and a horrible depression I was not in touch with. I was lost in an altered state, which is practically impossible to describe. The motor inside me was revved up for weeks on end. My brain was agitated and uncomfortable, and each day I worked hard to regain any sense of well-being I could, but it took two years before I succeeded.

The only activities I pursued were watching TV, sleeping, and doing meaningless jobs like dishes and cleaning. I found almost all social situations difficult, and as the months progressed, my fears multiplied. Eventually, my confidence plummeted. Losing track of my purpose seemed inevitable.

During this time, my psychiatrist prescribed an anti-psychotic that caused *one of my greatest breakthroughs.* I became relaxed and capable. Anxiety, sleep problems, depression, and mania disappeared.

One key factor in my experience with this illness is that, whenever medication was suggested or prescribed, *I took it.* Many people do not. They are no sooner on it than they want to get off. Sometimes, treatment for bipolar disorder becomes a battlefield. I feel frazzled if I don't take medication, but I still want to fix my condition fast. I believe I avoided being hospitalized my whole life because I was always medicated. There are many medications that help manage bipolar symptoms, and it is a far wiser course to take them than to muddle through without the medical breakthroughs that are available.

Time is on the side of anyone who developed bipolar after 1970, since that was when lithium was first introduced on the market. Prozac, a newer antidepressant, was widely prescribed in the United States by 1990. After 2003, new and more effective antipsychotics were developed and prescribed. I am so grateful that even better drugs will be discovered in my lifetime.

Sometimes, when times are tough, I tend to forget the other parts of my life that are really quite wonderful. As I write this, I am fifty-six years old. I have been dealing with bipolar since I was twelve. I am going to be dealing with it for the rest of my life, unless someone comes up with a cure. This is a permanent condition; I accept that. But I do not accept that it has to be a crippling condition that stops me in my tracks and leaves me immobilized. Every day there are small moments of happiness in my life. Major happiness occurs when I am stable—anchored, balanced, lasting, safe, and secure—when I forget I have bipolar disorder.

As I look back over my life, I sometimes find it difficult to believe all I have lived through: unexplainable physical and mental symptoms, endless trips to psychologists and psychiatrists, incorrect diagnoses, difficulties with vacations and moving, keeping it all a secret for so many years, and times when I wondered whether I would ever be able to lead a normal life. Yet, while all this was going on, I managed to get through college, hold down jobs, become an artist and musician, teach piano, maintain friendships, stay close to my family, remain married to the same man for thirty-one years, and raise two children.

When I began this book, I just wanted to tell my story and give others hope. My purpose then was to share the insights that would help people with bipolar disorder alleviate pain in their lives and find hope in their therapeutic plans. That is still my hope. Bipolar disorder is no rose garden; that is a fact. And while there are books out there written by a fortunate few who have suffered, found some magic elixir, and are living happily ever after, they are not the norm. The norm is more like the stock market: up, down, up, down, rarely flat.

The point is this: bipolar disorder is a condition we live with every day. Everybody has strengths and weaknesses. We need to be realistic, yet positive, about what we are capable of achieving. I am living proof of that.

In the end, we are in charge of creating and determining our own success.

Psychiatrists/Psychotherapists/Treatment

Name	Phone Number	Date First Seen	Date Last Seen

Support System

Name	Type of Support	Phone Number	E-Mail Address

Current Medications

Name Of Drug	Prescription Number	Date of Next Refillr	Physician's Name

Bipolar Triggers*

Trigger	Date Noticed	Type of Episode	Severity of Episode

* A trigger is an external cue or event that can set in motion an oncoming bipolar episode. Examples of triggers include sleep irregularities, poor nutrition, stress, and isolation. Definition excerpted from "Avoiding Triggers to Bipolar Episodes" by David E. Oliver.

www.ingramcontent.com/pod-product-compliance
Lightning Source LLC
Chambersburg PA
CBHW060613210326
41520CB00010B/1320